About the Editor – Nina Downes

Nina Downes has worked in the pharmaceutical industry for over 30 years in both blue chip and niche pharmaceutical companies as well as a large Contract Research Organisation. Over her long career she has gained extensive strategic and operational experience in all aspects of clinical research. Nina has held a number of high profile positions including Group Project Director, Head of Clinical Operations and Clinical Programme Director. She has a particular interest in the development and implementation of clinical strategies to support worldwide regulatory submissions and the challenge of successfully leading and motivating international multifunctional project teams. Nina's breadth of experience has been recognised by the award of an honorary lectureship in Clinical Research and she is currently director of Diamond Clinical Ltd, a company offering clinical research consultancy and training. Nina specialises in working with project teams facilitating the development of robust drug development plans and also in writing the clinical summaries for regulatory dossiers in CTD format.

Foreword

Clinical trials should be designed, conducted and analysed according to sound scientific principles to achieve their objectives; and should be reported appropriately. The essence of rational drug development is to ask important research questions and answer them with appropriate studies.

Pocock[15] states that there are three fundamental aspects of trial design which must be precisely defined at an early stage:

- Which patients are eligible?
- Which treatments are to be evaluated?
- How is each patient's response to be assessed?

A variety of study designs are used in clinical research. Different designs are appropriate in different circumstances and each can provide useful data. It is important to understand the advantages and disadvantages of each study type to enable the correct application of design to give appropriate and meaningful results.

The choice of design depends on why the trial is being conducted (e.g. for an MAA or for market support), the phase of the study, and the study endpoint. Whether it is a commercial or non-commercial study, Phase I, II, III or IV study, drug or device study, the basic principles remain the same. There should be a scientific and ethically sound question being asked and the design should be sufficient to answer the question being posed.

Designing a trial is a task that demands experience, statistical knowledge and time. In every trial, proof of efficacy is the primary aim with safety being of utmost importance. Demonstrating effectiveness is becoming increasingly important and therefore designs that demonstrate quality of life and pharmacoeconomics should be applied.

Evidence-based medicine (EBM) is the foundation for clinical practice and the results of properly conducted trials inform clinical practice. The strength of a study depends on its design; poorly designed trials may provide misleading information, which leads to inappropriate selection of treatments for patients.

Contents

About the Author – Sue Fitzpatrick ii

About the Editor – Nina Downes iii

Foreword.. iv

Chapter One – Introduction 1

Chapter Two – Approaches in design 2
Scientific approach in design. 2
The phases of a clinical development programme 3
  Phase I Most typical kind of study: human pharmacology 3
  Phase II Most typical kind of study: therapeutic exploratory 5
  Phase III Most typical kind of study: therapeutic confirmatory 5
  Phase IV Variety of studies: - therapeutic use 6
Trial design 6

Chapter Three – Considerations for study design 7
The elements of trial design. 7

Chapter Four – Patient population and indication
   for treatment.. 8
Patient population 8
Nature of the disease being treated 8
  Concurrent diseases and concomitant medication 9
  Influence of the indication on trial design 9

Chapter Five – Types of control 11
Choice of active control 11
The placebo-controlled trial 16

Chapter Six – Sources of bias, randomisation and blinding .. 19
Sources of bias 19
Randomisation 20
Levels of blinding 21

Chapter Seven – Types of trial design 24
Parallel and crossover designs. 24
  Parallel group. 24
Alternative trial designs 26
  Sequential design 26
  Factorial design 27
Within-patient design. 28

Chapter Eight – Duration of dosing and clinical methods.. .. 2?

Dosing 2

Methods of clinical measurement. 2

Chapter Nine – Other trial designs .. .. 3?

Epidemiology study designs. 3

Cohort studies 3

Case-control studies. 3

Outcomes research 3

Quality of life (QoL) 3

Pharmacoeconomic studies 3

Pharmacokinetic sampling/dose escalation/dose response 3

Repeated administration 3

Chapter Ten – Multicentre trials .. .. 3?

Designing a multicentre trial 3

Choice of comparator 3

The placebo-controlled trial 3

Patient population 3

Clinical measurement 38

Chapter Eleven – Evidence-based medicine (EBM) 39

Chapter Twelve – Reporting and publishing data .. .. 4?

Chapter Thirteen – Summary .. .. 4?

References .. .. 4?

Chapter One - Introduction

The foundation of clinical drug development is the clinical trial, and without a good design a clinical trial may fail to achieve its aim. Good trial design and conduct of clinical trials can provide the necessary knowledge for the generation of definitive answers about the effectiveness of new therapeutic approaches. In contrast, poorly designed or administered trials may provide misleading results, subject patients to unnecessary risk and waste considerable resources.

The multiple contexts within which biomedical research proceeds call for an array of research designs in order to assess scientific developments and advance clinical knowledge and treatment approaches. Any of a number of research designs may be appropriate for a clinical trial, depending on the context and circumstances of the research; however, every clinical trial must be scientifically sound and must incorporate important ethical principles regarding the treatment of research participants[1].

Before a clinical trial may proceed, it will undergo numerous reviews, including a review of the design and consideration of its applicability to the situation. A good trial design will ensure that the trial is given approval to proceed, from regulatory agencies, from ethics committees, from the Sponsor company and, of course, from the Investigator. A good design will ensure that the trial set-up is achievable, that the Investigator will recruit subjects and that the trial will be completed within the target timescale. The resulting report may then be presented (within a submission dossier) to regulatory agencies for approval of a drug, a new indication, or a new formulation.

Inappropriate or bad trial design may have consequences that are more far-reaching than the failure of one trial alone. One trial is part of a whole programme that supports the life of a drug. A failure in one part of that programme may lead, at best, to a delay in reaching targets or to the redesign of the programme, or at worst, to its cancellation. A major consequence of this is the cost, in money, time and other resources, and in the loss of a potentially useful drug, which may have been chosen for development in preference to another. Decisions made as a consequence of the result of a trial, *whether positive or negative*, must be taken with the confidence that the result is true. This is where the trial design is most important; any doubt as to the validity of the result indicates a problem in design. These considerations are encapsulated in the following sentence taken from section 6.4 of the International Conference on Harmonisation (ICH) good clinical practice (GCP) guideline[1]: 'The scientific integrity of the trial and the credibility of the data from the trial depend substantially on the trial design'.

The purpose of this monograph is to discuss the elements that must be considered in the design of a clinical trial.

Chapter Two - Approaches in design

Scientific approach in design

Clinical trials should be designed, conducted and analysed according to sound scientific principles to achieve their objectives; and should be reported appropriately. The essence of rational drug development is to ask relevant questions and answer them with appropriately designed studies. The primary objectives of any study should be clear and explicitly stated. Clinical studies can be classified according to when the study occurs during clinical development or, as shown in Table 1, by their objectives. (The illustrative examples are not intended to be exhaustive.) The logic behind serially conducted studies of a medicinal product is that the results of prior studies should be considered when reviewing the plan of later studies. Emerging data will frequently prompt a modification of the development strategy. For example, results of a therapeutic confirmatory study may suggest a need for additional human pharmacology studies.

Table 1. An approach to classifying clinical studies according to objective[2]

Type of study	Objective of study	Study examples
Human pharmacology	• Assess tolerance • Define/describe pharmacokinetics (PK) and pharmacodynamics (PD) • Explore drug metabolism and drug interactions • Estimate activity	• Dose-tolerance studies • Single and multiple dose PK and/or PD studies • Drug interaction studies
Therapeutic exploratory	• Explore use for the targeted indication • Estimate dosage for subsequent studies • Provide basis for confirmatory study design, endpoints, methodologies	• Earliest trials of relatively short duration in well-defined, narrow patient populations, using surrogate or pharmacological endpoints or clinical measures • Dose-response exploration studies

Therapeutic confirmatory	• Demonstrate/confirm efficacy • Establish safety profile • Provide an adequate basis for assessing the benefit/risk relationship to support licensing • Establish dose-response relationship	• Adequate, and well controlled studies to establish efficacy • Randomised parallel dose-response studies • Clinical safety studies • Studies of mortality/morbidity outcomes • Large simple trials • Comparative studies
Therapeutic use	• Refine understanding of benefit/risk relationship in general or special population and/or environments • Identify less common adverse reactions • Refine dosing recommendations	• Comparative effectiveness studies • Studies of mortality/morbidity outcomes • Studies of additional endpoints • Large simple trials • Pharmacoeconomic studies

The phases of a clinical development programme

The trials carried out in the development of a drug can be split into four temporal phases. These phases are helpful to gain a generalised view of drug development, and each phase requires a different approach to trial design. However, the definition of the phases is essentially arbitrary. It is also important to remember that the phases overlap. Some Phase I studies may still be ongoing when Phase II has started, for example drug-drug interactions or specialised pharmacokinetics in the elderly. One important point to note for those carrying out trials is that the EU Directives 2001/20/EC[3], 2005/28/EC[4] as well as ICH guidelines[1] apply to all phases.

While the content of the phase does not describe the design of a study, it can help determine the objectives of the phases. This definition based on objectives is in compliance with the ICH E8 guidelines[2] and the following definitions are also taken from that guideline:

Phase I Most typical kind of study: human pharmacology

Phase I starts with the initial administration of an investigational new drug (IND) into humans. Although human pharmacology studies are typically identified with Phase I, they may also be indicated at other points in the development sequence for example human pharmacology in paediatric populations must be carried out after adult studies. Studies in this phase of development usually have non-therapeutic objectives and may be conducted in healthy volunteer subjects or certain types of patients, e.g. patients with mild hypertension. Drugs with significant potential toxicity, e.g. cytotoxic drugs, are usually studied in patients. Studies in this phase can be open, baseline controlled or may use randomisation and blinding, to improve the validity of observations.

Studies conducted in Phase I typically involve one or a combination of the following aspects:

Estimation of initial safety and tolerability
The initial and subsequent administration of an investigational new drug into humans is usually intended to determine the tolerability of the dose range expected to be needed for later clinical studies and to determine the nature of adverse events or reactions that can be expected. These studies typically include both single and multiple dose administration.

Pharmacokinetics (PK)
Characterisation of a drug's absorption, distribution, metabolism, and excretion continues throughout the development of the drug. Their preliminary characterisation is an important goal of Phase I PK data and is particularly important when estimating the dose regimen or schedule to be used in later studies. Pharmacokinetics may be assessed via separate studies or as part of efficacy, safety and tolerance studies. Pharmacokinetic studies are particularly important to assess the clearance of the drug and to anticipate possible accumulation of parent drug or metabolites and potential drug-drug interactions. Some pharmacokinetic studies are conducted in later phases to answer more specialised questions such as the kinetics in the renally impaired. For many orally administered drugs, especially modified release products, the study of food effects on bioavailability is important. Obtaining pharmacokinetic information in sub-populations such as patients with impaired elimination (renal or hepatic failure), the elderly, children, women and ethnic subgroups should be considered. Drug-drug interaction studies are important for many drugs; these are generally performed in phases beyond Phase I but studies in animals and in vitro studies of metabolism and potential interactions may lead to doing such studies earlier.

Assessment of pharmacodynamics (PD)
Depending on the drug and the endpoint studied, pharmacodynamic studies and studies relating drug blood levels to response (PK/PD studies) may be conducted in healthy volunteer subjects or in patients with the target disease. In patients, if there is an appropriate measure, pharmacodynamic data can provide early estimates of activity and potential efficacy together with PK data and may guide the dosage and dose regimen in later studies.

Early measurement of drug activity
Preliminary studies of activity or potential therapeutic benefit may be conducted in Phase I as a secondary objective. Such studies are generally

The Institute of Clinical Research

performed in later phases but may be appropriate when drug activity is readily measurable with a short duration of drug exposure in patients at this early stage.

Phase II Most typical kind of study: therapeutic exploratory

Phase II is usually considered to start with the initiation of studies in which the primary objective is to explore therapeutic efficacy in patients. Initial therapeutic exploratory studies may use a variety of study designs, including concurrent controls and comparisons with baseline status. Subsequent trials are usually randomised and concurrently controlled to confirm the efficacy of the drug and its safety for a particular therapeutic indication. Studies in Phase II are typically conducted in a group of patients who are selected by relatively narrow criteria, leading to a relatively homogeneous population and are closely monitored. An important goal for this phase is to determine the dose(s) and regimen for Phase III trials. Early studies in this phase often utilise dose escalation designs (see ICH E4)[5] to give an early estimate of dose response and later studies may confirm the dose response relationship for the indication in question by using recognised parallel dose-response designs (could also be deferred to Phase III). Confirmatory dose-response studies may be conducted in Phase II or be part of the Phase III programme. Doses used in Phase II are usually but not always less than the highest doses used in Phase I. Additional objectives of clinical trials conducted in Phase II may include evaluation of potential study endpoints, therapeutic regimens (including concomitant medications) and target populations (e.g. mild versus severe disease) for further study in Phase II or III. These objectives may be served by exploratory analyses, examining subsets of data and by including multiple endpoints in trials which is a valid and important approach in these exploratory studies unlike the more formal approach required in the later confirmatory studies of Phase III.

Phase III Most typical kind of study: therapeutic confirmatory

Phase III is usually considered to begin with the initiation of studies in which the primary objective is to confirm therapeutic benefit. Studies in Phase III have a formal hypothesis and are designed to confirm the preliminary evidence accumulated in Phase II that a drug is safe and effective for use in the intended indication and recipient population. These studies are aimed at providing an adequate basis for marketing approval. Studies in Phase III may also further explore the dose-response relationship, or explore the drug's use in wider populations, in different stages of disease, or in combination with another drug. For drugs intended to be administered for long periods, trials involving extended exposure to the drug are ordinarily conducted in Phase III, although they may be started in Phase II. These studies carried out in Phase III complete the information needed to support adequate instructions for use of the drug (official product information).

Phase IV Variety of studies: - therapeutic use

Phase IV begins after drug approval. Therapeutic use studies go beyond the prior demonstration of the drug's safety, efficacy and dose definition. Studies in Phase IV are all studies (other than routine surveillance) performed after drug approval and related to the approved indication. They are studies that were not considered necessary for approval but are often important for optimising the drug's use. They may be of any type but should have valid scientific objectives. Commonly conducted studies include additional drug-drug interaction, dose-response or safety studies and studies designed to support use under the approved indication, e.g. mortality/morbidity studies, epidemiological studies.

Trial design

The design of any given clinical trial will be dependent on many contributing factors. The fundamental factor in the design is clearly the target indication, the influence that this will have on the objectives of the trial, the options for clinical measurement, and the circumstances in which the trial is to be carried out. Bearing in mind that the individual trial is part of a larger clinical development plan, some of the influencing factors such as target population, primary endpoints etc. may already be defined, and there may be standards set by the programme plan that must be included in the design. These must be considered where appropriate.

Chapter Three - Considerations for study design

In this chapter the objective is to describe the elements that make up a clinical trial, and to suggest how these should be considered when designing a trial, or reviewing a design. The person designing a trial is reliant upon information from many sources: the statistician, the regulatory experts, the clinical trial supplies/packaging group, the data processing group, the preclinical pharmacologists, the medical experts and the Investigators.

The elements of trial design

Although this monograph is too short to provide an account of all possible clinical trial designs, Table 2 summarises those elements of trial design that will be considered in some detail. It is important to obtain input from all available sources, and in particular, to be aware that not all designs are appropriate to all situations. A particular therapeutic area or study phase of development may have specific trial designs that have become standards.

Table 2. Summary of elements to be considered in clinical trial design.

Indication for treatment
Patient population
• Indication being treated
• Concurrent diseases
• Concomitant medication
Types of control
• Active control
• Placebo control
Sources of bias
Randomisation
Levels of blinding
Types of trial design
• Parallel
• Crossover
• Other trial designs
Duration of dosing
Methods of clinical measurement

Chapter Four - Patient population and indication for treatment

Patient population

The patient population from which the study participants will be drawn must be carefully defined to avoid the bias that derives from a non-defined, perhaps Investigator-specific, selection strategy. In early Phase II the entry criteria for a study may be very restrictive, and throughout the development programme, these criteria will be adjusted to be more inclusive to reflect the intended target population as the drug's characteristics are discovered. For example, Phase I trials may have studied healthy volunteers, probably with a restricted age range usually between 18 and 45 years. As further studies are completed in older (and possibly in younger) subjects, the newer study protocols may be extended to include these age groups. By the end of Phase III, the studies should include a population that is representative of the wider patient population, who will potentially receive the licensed drug; the trial results should have generality. The protocol should define clearly which subjects are eligible for entry into a study, so that the differences between groups may be reliably ascribed to treatment differences, and not to variability between subjects.

The following are some of the points to consider when preparing the inclusion and exclusion criteria:

- Nature and history of the disease being treated
- Concurrent diseases
- Concurrent medication.

In the effort to achieve uniformity in the population of study participants, there must always be consultation with the Investigators who are to carry out the trial. Otherwise there is a risk of limiting the selection criteria to such an extent that the trial may not be feasible.

Nature of the disease being treated

Variability is inherent within any population or sub-population. In a study of an antihypertensive therapy, simply enrolling any subject with elevated blood pressure will introduce a wide range of variability into the trial. This may have consequences for the response that is being measured, as this will also be variable. Expressed in terms of the actual blood pressure, subjects with severe hypertension could display improvement of a greater magnitude than those with mild hypertension. Therefore, the disease severity should be specified. In particular, terms such as mild, moderate or severe must be clearly and objectively defined in the protocol. Using the example of hypertension, this may be expressed in terms of a diastolic blood pressure between x mmHg and y mmHg. Continuing with this example, caution must be exercised to ensure that information is gathered for all three grades of severity to avoid unnecessarily limiting the final registration of the drug to one of these categories only. This can be done in one study by stratifying for severity or separate studies for each severity may be appropriate. However, there may be cases where the conclusion is that the new agent is an effective antihypertensive drug only in patients, for example, with severe hypertension. A large variability in disease severity will necessitate a greater sample size. Other sources of variability due to disease may derive from the time since disease onset or diagnosis, and response to previous treatment.

Concurrent diseases and concomitant medication
It is unlikely that the patient population suffering from the target disease will present with no concurrent diseases. This fact will undoubtedly affect the interpretation of trial results and therefore must be considered in the criteria for selecting study participants. In the early phases the decision to include or exclude subjects with specific diseases will be based on preclinical pharmacology, the knowledge base can then be extended in the light of the results of Phase I and Phase II trials.

Concurrent diseases may influence the efficacy and safety of the drug through, for example, metabolic interaction, but the necessity for medication to treat a concurrent disease may confound the interpretation of the result. Hence, concurrent diseases and concomitant medication need to be considered together.

Influence of the indication on trial design
Some elements that are considered when designing a trial will be influenced by the natural history of the disease being treated. For example, the onset and progression of the disease will affect the duration of the trial, the timing of each subject's treatment, and the number and timing of assessments.

A neat classification of disease might be between acute and chronic, each having implications for trial design. Acute indications, for example infections or musculoskeletal injuries, will require a short treatment period, and during that period it is expected that a cure (or at least an improvement) would be effected. These types of disease also display spontaneous remission within a certain time after onset. Additionally, the signs and symptoms are not constant, and indeed may initially increase in severity. Therefore, the known profile of the disease may dictate that the study treatment period is one week, that subjects should enter the study within one day of onset, and that assessments be carried out daily for the first four days, to detect any signs of efficacy in the early stages. In comparison, the signs and symptoms of some chronic diseases will be stable over long periods of time. This may dictate, for example, a study of six months duration, with monthly assessments carried out for efficacy. (More frequent assessments at the start of the treatment period will be necessary in early phase studies to monitor safety).

The Institute of Clinical Research

This rather simplistic approach to chronic disease may be confounded when study participants are already receiving treatment that may necessitate a wash-out period. Any withdrawal of previous therapy must be carefully considered, so as not to destabilise the subject without clinical justification. If a wash-out period is used, the trial design should incorporate repeat assessments of the variable under study (e.g. blood pressure) to provide a stable baseline against which to assess efficacy.

The nature of the disease may, however, dictate that withdrawal of any current therapy is not clinically justifiable. There are several ways to continue clinical development despite this hurdle. The first is to use only subjects who are newly diagnosed with the condition. This will mean that the number of subjects available for the study will be reduced compared with the total population suffering from that disease. One implication is a longer trial and another is the need to access a large population from which to recruit such subjects. Alternatively, the need to withdraw treatment can be avoided by designing a trial where the test treatment is added to the current treatment. This implies that current therapy is inadequate and that there is still measurable improvement to be gained, either in terms of efficacy or safety. This type of add-on trial may be used, for example, in epilepsy. There is a need for adequate knowledge about the potential for interaction between treatments. In this situation a placebo may be the most appropriate comparator. Following a trial that proves efficacy and safety of the combination treatment, it may be appropriate to design trials that investigate the potential for decreasing the dose of the standard medication, while still maintaining efficacy. This is a particularly appealing approach when the standard therapy has an adverse event profile that is clinically undesirable. This type of trial is frequently referred to as a 'sparing' trial, and examples appear in the use of systemic corticosteroids, anti-rejection treatments, and narcotic analgesics.

Some diseases may be cyclical in nature, exhibiting periods of exacerbation and remission. One example in this category is rheumatoid arthritis, and many clinical trials featuring this condition are described in the literature. The anticipated length of the cycle between the two extremes of disease will influence the time at which subjects can be entered into the study in order to ensure a standardised baseline population. It will also influence the treatment period within the study because the remission of the disease itself may inflate the apparent treatment effect.

Some diseases are seasonal, one obvious example being hayfever. To complete a study within one season will require careful planning, with particular consideration given to sample size and the necessity for many centres. A backup plan to roll over to the other hemisphere could be considered.

Chapter Five - Types of control

To enable a robust conclusion to be made from the results of a scientific study, there must be a control group. The purpose of the control group is to provide a yardstick against which to measure the efficacy and safety of the drug under investigation. The control may be an untreated group or a group receiving an active treatment (which could even be standard care) or a placebo.

ICH E10[6] classifies controls on the basis of two critical attributes:

(1) the type of treatment used and (2) the method of determining who will be in the control group.

The type of control treatment may be any of the following five:

- Placebo
- No treatment
- Different dose or regimen of the study treatment
- A different active treatment
- External (historical) control groups.

Historical controls are employed in retrospective studies, which utilise data from medical history, either from the literature or from records of the same institution or from a previous but similar trial. These studies are mostly used in Phase IV, the prime example being the case-control study.

Most studies are carried out prospectively. In a prospective study the control group is studied as part of the trial in question; all subjects are entered into the study over the same time interval and experience the same conditions of treatment with either the study drug or control treatment. The comparator group therefore 'controls' sources of variability due to the situation, so that any differences between the groups can be attributed with confidence to the difference between the treatments. The situation in which the study is carried out may introduce variability due to geographical location or the season of the year. Alternatively, outcome may be affected by elements of the social or political environment.

Choice of active control

Although placebos are a frequently used control for clinical trials, it is increasingly commonplace to compare an experimental intervention to an existing established effective treatment. These types of studies are called *active-control* (or positive control) *studies*, which can take two forms—*a superiority trial*, in which the question is whether the new drug will be superior to the active control, and an *equivalence* or non-inferiority *trial*, in which the question is whether the new drug will be equivalent to (equivalence trial) or at least as good as (non-inferior to) the active control. Active-controlled trials are often extremely useful in cases in which it would be unethical to give participants a placebo because doing so would pose undue risk to their health or well-being. In an active-control study, participants are randomly assigned to the experimental intervention or to an active-control treatment. Such trials are often double blinded, but this is not always possible. Many oncology studies are considered impossible to blind because of the variable regimens, different routes of administration, and range of toxicities involved. In a study in which an active control is used, it may be difficult to determine whether the active control or the experimental intervention had an effect unless the effects of the treatments are obvious or a placebo control is included. For example, because the natural history of depression varies from patient to patient and it is often difficult to prove that a standard treatment has had an effect, studies of anti-depressants usually include both an active control arm and a placebo control arm, often unequally randomised because differences versus placebo are expected to be greater and therefore require fewer patients which means that fewer patients are exposed to placebo.

ICH efficacy guideline E10 Choice of Control Group and Related Issues[6] provides guidelines for choosing comparators. Although trials using any of the control groups described and discussed in the guideline may be useful and acceptable in clinical trials that serve as the basis for marketing approval in at least some circumstances, they are not equally appropriate or useful in every case. The general approach to selecting the type of control is outlined in Figure 1, and Table 3.

Table 3. Usefulness of specific concurrent control types in various situations

Type of control								
Trial objective	Placebo	Active non-inferiority	Active superiority	Dose response (D/R)	Placebo + Active	Placebo + D/R	Active + D/R	Placebo + Active + D/R
Measure 'absolute' effect size	Y	N	N	N	Y	Y	N	Y
Show existence of effect	Y	P	Y	Y	Y	Y	Y	Y
Show dose-response relationship	N	N	N	Y	N	Y	Y	Y
Compare therapies	N	P	Y	N	Y	N	P	Y

Y=yes, N=no, P=possible, depending on whether there is historical evidence of sensitivity to drug effects D/R = dose response = different doses of the drug.

Figure 1. Choosing the Concurrent Control for Demonstrating Efficacy

This figure shows the basic logic for choosing the control group, the decision may depend on the available drugs.

| Is there proven effective treatment? | NO → | **Options**
• Placebo control with design modifications[1], if appropriate
• Dose-response control
• Active control seeking to show superiority of test drug to active control
• No-treatment control with design modifications[1], if appropriate
• Any combination of the above controls |

YES ↓

| Is the proven effective treatment life-saving or known to prevent irreversible morbidity? | YES → | **Options**
• Active control, superiority, or non-inferiority if there is historical evidence of sensitivity to drug effect
• Placebo control with appropriate design modifications[1] (e.g. add-on study)
• Dose-response control (limited cases) |

NO ↓

| Is there historical evidence of sensitivity to drug effects for an appropriately designed and conducted trial | NO → | **Options**
• Placebo control with design modifications[1], if appropriate
• Dose-response control
• Active control showing superiority to control
• No-treatment control with design modifications[1], if appropriate
• Active and placebo controls |

YES ↓

| | YES → | **Options**
• Placebo control with design modifications[1], if appropriate
• Dose-response control
• Active control seeking showing superiority to control
• Active and placebo controls
• Active control non-inferiority |

Table 3 describes the usefulness of specific types of control groups, and Figure 1 provides a decision tree for choosing among different types of control groups. Although Table 3 and Figure 1 focus on the choice of control to demonstrate efficacy, some designs also allow comparisons of test and control agents. The choice of control can be affected by the availability of therapies and by medical practices in specific regions. The potential usefulness of the principal types of control (placebo, active, and dose response) in specific situations and for specific purposes is shown in Table 3.

The choice of comparator for the control group is greatly influenced by, and greatly influences, trial design. This, combined with the constraints imposed by the characteristics of the test compound, makes selection of the comparator a question of vital importance when considering the design of a study. The following are some of the points, both theoretical and practical, to consider when choosing the comparator:

1. *Objective of the study.* In simple terms, the objective of most studies is to investigate the efficacy and safety of a compound under test. In order to maintain clarity of design it is paramount that every study has one primary objective that is stated in the protocol. In cases where efficacy has not yet been established, it may be that a placebo is the most appropriate comparator. A comparison against a non-pharmacologically active compound will undoubtedly provide the answer to questions of efficacy. However, the use of placebo is fraught with ethical issues and practical trial management issues, the comparative importance of which will depend on the disease being treated and the treatments currently available. The use of placebo will be addressed separately later.

   Assuming that the compound has been shown to possess efficacy, the objectives of later studies (Phase III onwards) will be to compare the extent of efficacy and safety with that of currently used therapies. These studies will be used as a major component of the regulatory submission, and therefore input from the regulatory department is most important. These colleagues will be able to provide information as to what is accepted as the best current treatment against which all new treatments must be compared as well as the latest regulatory guidelines and thinking on clinical trial design in a particular therapeutic area. As a further source of valuable input the marketing department or business information will provide information as to the most widely prescribed current treatment. It will be valuable for future marketing to have a comparison against such treatment(s). This means that although the stated scientific objective of any study will be an assessment of efficacy and safety, in order to maximise the benefit of a study to the development programme, these secondary objectives must be considered when selecting a comparator.

   The objective of the study therefore is linked to the phase of the development programme.

2. *Countries where the study is to be carried out.* This is an area where thorough research is needed, particularly in multi-centre, multinational or even global studies. The vagaries of the regulatory process may mean that a drug that has been suggested as a potential comparator may not be approved for sale or, if approved, may not be marketed in countries scheduled for participation in the clinical trial. In these cases there may be regulatory obstacles to running the study in that country. A further source of variation between countries can be found in the different formulations and dosing instructions that are registered in different countries. This may be particularly true for older drugs that have many generic forms or older non standardised marketing licences.

3. *Registration status of the potential comparator.* For the reasons stated above, when discussing the objective of the study, regulatory and marketing

considerations suggest that it is most productive to choose an active comparator that is established and marketed. This will also have practical benefits.

To use two unlicensed drugs in a study increases the complexity of set-up for two reasons. From the regulatory point of view, full information about both drugs would have to be submitted to the licensing authority in an IMPD (Investigational Medicinal Product Dossier) and it would be highly unlikely that a competitor company would make their preclinical information available to another company. From the practical point of view, it would be very difficult to obtain supplies for use in a comparative study from the manufacturer of a future potential competitor.

Included under this heading is the status of the drug in terms of exclusivity. While a patent is still current for any drug, it is likely that the drug will be available only from the original manufacturer or its licensees. Since the ideal study design may be considered to be double-blind, and marketed formulations are often identifiable, perhaps by unique markings on a tablet, it is difficult to ensure a double-blind supply of medication. Sometimes a simple encapsulation of a tablet may be possible, but any manipulation (e.g. grinding a tablet to fill a capsule) will mean not only extra work for the clinical trial supplies department but also, as a minimum, dissolution studies to ensure that this manipulation has not affected the characteristics of the formulation such as bioavailability. Blinding might necessitate the use of a double-dummy design. Placebos matching the active treatment must be obtained, and this will undoubtedly be from the patent holder and will take time and sometimes mean revealing your protocol!

When a patent is no longer current, generic forms will be available and manufacturers will frequently supply their active formulation with matching placebos, perhaps more quickly than in the on-patent situation.

Consideration of these practical factors must necessarily be accommodated when designing the study, as delays may mean that the trial fails to achieve its schedule and this will have implications for the whole development programme. A balance must be struck between time schedule to do the study and target time for the file to be submitted.

4. *Dosing regimens of the potential comparator.* It has already been stated that for a study to have value for both registration and marketing, the study drug should be compared with a known and established active treatment. The active comparator should be used in the way in which it is known to be effective. Therefore, it is not advisable to use a dosing regimen different from that registered or in common use. To do so would create specific problems that would need to be taken into account in the trial design. Examples of such problems might be that the comparator has a once-daily dosing regimen while the test drug has a twice-daily regimen;

alternatively, one of the two may be formulated to be long-acting or slow-release. Differences in dosing frequency may reflect a difference in the pharmacokinetic properties of the two drugs. A further, more complex, situation related to pharmacokinetics might arise if one of the drugs has a very long or a very short half-life. This may affect how a subject is withdrawn from the drug, a factor that is of particular significance in a crossover trial where a wash out period is required between treatments.

Dosing instructions for established drugs will reflect their pharmacodynamic activity; for example, withdrawal of the drug may have to be gradual to avoid precipitating a worsening of symptoms. In designing the trial so that its level of blinding is maintained, clear instructions must be included to take account of issues such as these.

5. *Marketing input.* The sales and marketing department will offer input as to the most appropriate comparator for its purposes. In some cases there may be reasons for carrying out trials late in Phase III to allow comparison with drugs that are specific to only one country: treatment of some diseases shows a marked specificity to individual countries.

The placebo-controlled trial

A placebo-controlled study is a study where subjects are randomly assigned to a placebo. When there is no established (standard) treatment for a disease, the Food and Drug Administration (FDA) 21 CFR part 314[8] states that a placebo control is often the design of choice. Indeed, a placebo controlled clinical trial is generally considered to be the most scientifically valid study. However, if a treatment exists that has been shown to be effective, it is unethical to use a placebo, particularly if the illness is life-threatening.

The ethical issues raised by the use of a pharmacologically inactive control have to be considered.

For some clinical trials in certain disease areas (e.g. non serious diseases), the decision regarding the appropriateness of using a placebo is not problematic. It is generally accepted that when no established intervention exists to treat or prevent the condition being studied, it is ethically acceptable to give the control group a placebo. Another argument in favour of the use of placebo controls has been made in the context of research conducted in a developing country. Many researchers have contended that the research question must be defined differently in a setting in which health care resources are limited and participants do not have access to established effective treatments outside of the research context. Some have advocated that in these cases, the measurement of absolute efficacy of a new and potentially more affordable and available intervention is a more relevant research question for the host country than the comparison of a new intervention to an established effective treatment already available elsewhere.

On the other hand, many experts believe that a placebo-controlled trial would not be ethical if an established effective treatment that is known to prevent serious harm, such as death or irreversible injury, is available and can be provided. In such a situation comparison with placebo would be possible if both the new treatment and placebo is added to standard care.

Yet, there are some who criticise the use of placebo controls even in cases in which risks to participants are low. One argument against the use of placebos was published in the Declaration of Helsinki: Ethical Principles for Medical Research Involving Human Subjects[9], which states that "in any medical study, every patient, including those of a control group, if any, should be assured of the best proven diagnostic and therapeutic method".

The recent revision of the Declaration of Helsinki[10] attempts to resolve the debate about placebos by recommending "the benefits, risks, burdens and effectiveness of a new method should be tested against those of the best current prophylactic, diagnostic and therapeutic methods. This does not exclude the use of placebo, or no treatment, in studies where no proven prophylactic, diagnostic or therapeutic method exists". Certain criticisms about this provision remain, principally that it makes it very difficult, if not impossible, to conduct placebo-controlled trials when such trials may be the only method of addressing the health needs of a particular population.

Ethics review committees will rightfully exercise their judgment in assessing research designs that employ a placebo control. In situations in which the best scientific design is not ethically acceptable, it may be necessary to reconsider the primary research question and to choose one for which an ethically acceptable design can be proposed, or it may be necessary to accept the fact that ethical constraints can create limitations to obtaining scientific knowledge.

We will address some of the practical issues that are prerequisites for designing a placebo-controlled trial. Essentially, all these points must be considered for any trial, but they are particularly pertinent to designs involving a placebo control, and include:

- Withdrawals due to inadequate efficacy

- Selection of an appropriate population of trial subjects

- Sample size.

The ideal placebo is a formulation of the excipients from the test medication, 'and will be identical in appearance to the test medication'[8].

Treatment with placebo is sometimes efficacious (the so-called placebo effect), and can also produce significant adverse reactions. The extent of these effects varies between different indications. For example, in patients with angina, exercise tolerance has been shown to increase by about 10%

in the placebo group compared with 22% in the active treatment group[11]. In contrast, in patients with diabetes, placebo produced no effect on blood glucose levels. Placebo-induced adverse effects also vary between indication groups. Weihrauch and Gauler[11] conclude that placebo treatment cannot be considered as 'non-treatment' and that the effects of placebo must be known before the effects of active treatment can be assessed.

The placebo effect is particularly apparent when the clinical measurement is subjective. Hrobjartsson[9] is sceptical about the 'powerful placebo' but acknowledges a significant effect of placebo analgesia over no treatment. This is illustrated clearly by trials of analgesics in which it can be expected that about 25% of the placebo group will record some measure of pain relief following a single dose[12]. This finding highlights two points. First, why was the placebo group included? It must be assumed that this finding is due to the placebo effect plus the background rate of 'recovery' against which the test treatment is to be judged. Second, it also means that 75% of placebo patients do not achieve any pain relief, and so the study design must specify how those subjects will be handled.

In preparing the design, clear instructions must be given to the Investigator (who has to treat the subject) on how that subject should be treated in the clinic, including specification of any rescue or escape medication. This will depend on how the subject's results will be analysed statistically. In the example of the single-dose analgesic trial, in the event of withdrawal due to inadequate pain relief, the result of the last pain assessment (i.e. at the time of withdrawal when pain severity was great) might be carried over for all subsequent assessment times, and this assumes a worst-case scenario for the analysis. Alternatively, the time to relief of symptoms may be an appropriate primary endpoint.

The Investigator could therefore be instructed to withdraw the subject from the study, and the subject will be given the most appropriate standard treatment. The net result of including such substitution will be that the subject's data will contribute a value of 'no response' to the analysis of the placebo group.

In gathering information to assist in designing the study, one of the most valuable pieces of information for the statistician will concern the level of difference between treatments that will be considered as clinically relevant. Since the placebo response may be considered to be the least expected, the sample size required to demonstrate efficacy of the test treatment will be smaller than for a comparison with another active treatment. Accurate characterisation of the placebo response will include an assessment of the spontaneous improvement of the disease, for which reference may be made to previous clinical trials or epidemiology studies.

Chapter Six - Sources of bias, randomisation and blinding

For a trial to make a credible contribution to the governing clinical development plan, the result must not be biased by any outside influence. All clinical trials should be designed to avoid bias so that the result achieved is clearly representative of the drug's effect. Ensuring that the chosen study design avoids various forms of bias and generates data that can answer the scientific questions being asked can be difficult.

Sources of bias

It is important in any trial to minimise the sources of bias. The most frequently used mechanisms for eliminating bias are through the use of control treatments, definition of the study population, randomisation and blinding.

A major cause of bias in the interpretation of a drug's activity appears when the people involved in the clinical trial hold preconceived expectations of that activity. A precept required at the outset of any trial is that the Investigator assumes impartiality, and this is embodied in the adoption of a null hypothesis that the trial will reveal no difference[13]. This 'therapeutic equipoise' should be held by the Investigator, the subject and the Sponsor's representatives. However, the absolute requirement for sharing all known information about the drug at the time of establishing a trial is likely to unbalance this impartiality.

The way that this will introduce bias may be reflected in the Investigator's choice of subjects to be treated with the trial product. For example, concerns about a potential adverse effect may lead the Investigator to select a study population that may have a lower risk of experiencing the adverse effect in question. In the case where an Investigator is unconvinced of efficacy, the population selected may be those subjects who exhibit a less severe form of the target disease.

In the case of a comparative study, an Investigator may select which subject will receive which drug, perhaps on grounds similar to those cited in the previous paragraph. Such a selection strategy may yield results that cannot be transferred to a real patient population. This could be particularly dangerous if the basis for selection is not documented.

Another source of bias relates to the nature of the target indication. Many diseases are cyclical in nature, having periods of flare-up and remission. One such example is rheumatoid arthritis. Other diseases that are self-limiting will improve even without treatment, for example, certain infections or injuries. The result of a trial for a treatment of such diseases will be biased by the stage of the disease at which the treatment is introduced. This makes it difficult to separate the effect of the test treatment from the natural history of the disease.

The Institute of Clinical Research

The choice and method of use of clinical measurements is also a potential source of bias. This is illustrated particularly where the measurement method is subjective, for example, in the assessment of pain. The individual subject's response to a question about a sensation will be influenced by the way in which the question is asked and by the choice of words available. Both these influences may be affected by the observer's and the subject's preconceived idea of the trial or treatment, and may be further compounded by existing relationships between the interviewer and the subject. A willingness to please can bias the result towards efficacy, or some other concern may lead to a more negative response.

Randomisation

Two foundation stones for the development of a trial's design have been established. A control group will be included, and the study population has been defined. Within that definition of subject characteristics, however, there will still be variability. For example, ages may range from 18 to 65 years, both men and women may be included, and more than one grade of severity may be allowed. This will provide an opportunity for the introduction of bias because an Investigator may consider that all 18- to 30-year-olds should receive treatment A. This would mean that the two treatment groups may not be comparable, i.e. any difference in efficacy or safety may be due to more than just the drug. To overcome this selection bias, subjects are allocated to treatment using a method called randomisation. In a randomised trial successive subjects are assigned to a treatment in a predetermined but random manner.

The most common practice when randomising subjects is simple randomisation which assigns equal numbers to each treatment group. However, there are situations where unequal randomisation may be appropriate[14]. By allocating more of the subjects to a new treatment, more experience of its effects can be gained, particularly if the comparator is a well-known standard. A further advantage is that fewer subjects are needed for a placebo/active comparison than for an active/active comparison.

In cases where there are differences in the nature of the disease, for example, relating to severity or site, there may be different responses to treatment. Randomisation should ensure that each treatment group contains a sample of subjects with the same extent of variability as the defined population. However, if a marked degree of difference in the response is predicted, *stratification* can be employed.

This means that separate randomisation lists are prepared for each of the different disease categories or strata, so that there will be an equal number of subjects receiving each of the treatments within each of the disease categories[13]. Examples of the use of stratification might be to separate subjects with mild or severe pain in an analgesic trial, where the response might be different, or to separate subjects with a first or second renal transplant in a study of an immunosuppressant drug because the risk factors for rejection might be different. Each stratum may then be analysed separately, if deemed appropriate. Advice is required from the medical expert to identify the relevant prognostic factors and then a statistician must ensure that use of stratification is appropriate.

In a useful review, Kernan[15] concludes that stratification is important in small trials in which known clinical factors may have a major influence on prognosis, hence affecting treatment outcome, and it's also useful in large trials when interim analyses are planned with small numbers of subjects. Another method that can be used to produce treatment groups that are well matched for several variables is adaptive randomisation or *minimisation*. Minimisation takes the approach of assigning subjects to treatment groups in order to minimise the differences between the treatment groups on selected prognostic factors. The method starts with a simple randomisation method for the first several subjects and then adjusts the chance of allocating a new patient to a particular treatment based on existing imbalances in those prognostic factors. Let us compare treatment A and treatment B with age as a prognostic factor <20 age in years or >20 age in years. If treatment A has more <20 than >20 then the allocation scheme is such that the next few <20 patients are more likely to be randomised to treatment B. This method is used when there are many prognostic factors to be considered so patient allocation is then based on the aim of balancing the subtotals for each level of each factor[16]. With the increasing availability of interactive randomisation systems via telephone or the Internet, sophisticated randomisation methods may be easily incorporated into clinical trial designs.

Levels of blinding

An *open* study is one in which both the subject and the Investigator are aware of the identity of the treatment given.

Open studies are appropriate where knowledge of the treatment received does not enable the subject or Investigator to influence the results of the study, for example, in pharmacokinetic studies. In a pharmacokinetic study in a First Time in Man study or Phase I trial the objective is to ascertain if the drug is safe and what the likely acceptable dose is. Not all Phase I studies are open as there still could be sources of bias in a Phase I study. For example, if you conduct a study in a six-bed ward of a Phase I unit and a light fitting flickers all day, it is very likely that the subjects will develop a headache. If we have no control group the headache would be attributed to the treatment under study. If we compared it against placebo however and subjects given placebo also develop headaches then we cannot conclude that it is treatment induced.

In a comparative study, however, when treatment is given in an open manner, the sources of bias are many. The subject or the Investigator may feel eager to please and their assessment of efficacy and reports of adverse events may favour the new treatment and introduce assessment bias. Conversely, despite informed consent, they may have a negative attitude to the new drug and provide an entirely negative opinion. The drop-out rate might also be biased because subjects and Investigators may be more cautious with a new treatment than with the familiar standard.

Open studies may be used for pilot studies to give justification for developing larger randomised controlled trial (RCT) studies at a reduced cost, as they are simple to conduct. There are no development costs of a placebo or blinding procedures. Unlike an RCT there is no need to have large numbers as we are only looking to see if the pharmacokinetics and safety profile of the drug is acceptable to develop further. In fact an open trial in a single patient case study, or with more patients a case series study, could be conducted.

A case study is a brief description of a single case that an observer feels should be brought to the attention of colleagues, such as an unusual episode of poisoning or an atypical rash developing after administration of a new drug.

Case series are several case reports of similar observations or procedures that may be grouped together usually in consecutive patients. Case series may be an important way to establish a new surgical procedure. The advantage of this type of study is that it is simple to perform and can be written up and published rapidly. The disadvantage is that there is limited insight about the disease or treatment efficacy and retrospective case series may contain incomplete data.

Although comparative safety even in the long-term is the gold standard, some Therapeutic Confirmatory (Phase III) studies are also designed as open label if long-term safety data is required, e.g. in chronic diseases such as rheumatoid arthritis where the treatment will be used continuously or intermittently for a number of years.

An example of an open label study is the 'Leflunomide in the Treatment of Active Rheumatoid Arthritis (RA) in Everyday Clinical Use'[17]. This study investigated for the first time, the efficacy and safety profile of leflunomide 20mg daily in ambulatory RA patients in typical settings. This is of importance, as the existing body of evidence of leflunomide therapy is mainly derived from the artificial setting of a clinical development programme[17].

Sometimes it is unethical to perform an RCT. If we were comparing surgery and non-surgery would it be ethical to carry out a pretend operation, i.e. cut open the subject then close them back up without undertaking the surgical procedure?

To avoid these biases, the majority of clinical trials are carried out in a 'blind' manner. There are two primary levels of blinding: a *single-blind* study is one in which the subject or the Investigator does not know which treatment has been administered; and a *double-blind* study is one in which neither the subject nor the Investigator knows which treatment has been given. A *double dummy* may be required where there is a difference in formulation or dosing regimes to be compared. The double-blind design is generally considered the preferable type of study. In designing such a study it must be remembered that there may be decision points for which the Investigator in clinical practice would need to know the identity of all drugs administered. Contingency must be built in to accommodate this, either by disclosing the treatment by means of code breaks or by providing some type of decision tree. An example of such a contingency in the event of failure might be the use of a specified rescue medication that is known not to interact with either of the blinded treatments, to avoid breaking the blind.

Maintenance of the blind nature of the study is vital to preserve the impartiality of the Investigator. It is at the study design stage that full consideration must be given as to how this blind will be maintained, especially if there are differences in the presentation of the various treatments. A further level of blinding may be appropriate, in addition to the subjects and the Investigators and their staff. It is conceivable that representatives of the Sponsor may unwittingly influence the Investigator because they are aware of the treatment allocations. This may become apparent to the Investigator because of a particular focus at monitoring visits. It is therefore appropriate that monitoring staff should not become aware of treatment allocation, and it may be necessary to consider the use of an independent committee to monitor safety reports.

Chapter Seven - Types of trial design

The most frequently used designs for prospective clinical trials are the *parallel* study and the *crossover* study, although many other alternative designs are possible[18]. It is helpful to review the available literature of published trials carried out in the area of clinical interest to establish what alternatives are applicable. Several textbooks also contain descriptions of clinical trial designs[17].

Parallel and crossover designs

The two main trial designs, the crossover study and the parallel group study have been described in the Clinical Trial Protocol monograph[14] but are reproduced here as they are the most widely used designs.

Parallel group' design: each subject receives only one of the treatments for a predetermined time. The responses in groups of subjects are then compared

Parallel group

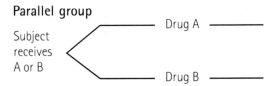

Parallel group designs are usually the design of choice for most therapeutic exploratory and therapeutic confirmatory (Phase II and III) studies intended for regulatory submissions, where an objective scientific assessment of the relative efficacy and safety of two or more treatments is required. Subjects enter the trial and are randomised to one of the treatments to be compared, and the between treatment group responses are analysed. These trials are often conducted blind, especially where the primary endpoint is a subjective one. If there are two treatments to be compared then this is referred to as a two-arm parallel group study, three treatments will mean three-arms etc.

In a parallel study, each subject is assigned to receive one or other of the treatments, and the subjects are studied 'in parallel'. The advantage of this design is that bias can be kept to a minimum (e.g. no sequence effects) and the disadvantage is that variability between patients and therefore the treatment groups can affect the results. This between patient variability can be accounted for by using an accurate standard deviation (SD) in the sample size calculation, which usually minimises this disadvantage.

In a crossover design, each subject receives one treatment then crosses over to receive the other treatment. The response within each subject is then compared.

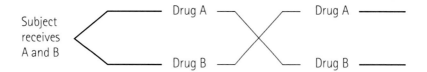

The advantage of a crossover study is that each subject receives all treatments to be compared, and the variation of the measurement is within each subject. This will be less than in a parallel group trial, where the variation of measurement is between groups of subjects as each subject only gets one treatment. The disadvantage of the crossover study is that it can only be used for efficacy trials if the disease is such that an adequate washout period can be included to avoid a different baseline when the second treatment is given (the effect of the first treatment could be carried over). In order to ensure this, the disease must be stable and the washout period long enough to ensure no carry over effect. This sort of design, therefore, is not used in diseases where there is marked disease progression, or in studies of diseases where it would not be ethical to withhold treatment, or if the safety of the subject would be at risk during washout, or the washout period would be too long to be practical (e.g. acute studies on antibiotics).

Crossover studies are often used in episodic conditions such as migraine where the subject returns to baseline values after each episode. Crossover designs are used in Phase I studies to evaluate the effect of food or drug interactions and in later phase studies destined for marketing use, where the aim of the study is to assess subject acceptability of the treatments being compared. As every subject receives every treatment, acceptability of use can be compared.

The choice of one of these two designs over the other demands careful consideration. Selection of the crossover design may be appealing because each subject acts as his/her own control, and in the context of clinical treatment this may be helpful in identifying which treatment is best for that particular subject. However, the application of that result to the general population cannot be extrapolated from the results of that particular subject's individual crossover trial. Nevertheless, crossover designs may be excellent models for demonstrating efficacy in Phase II studies, or for investigating phenomena such as drug interactions.

One practical issue to consider is subject (and perhaps Investigator) compliance with the protocol. A typical crossover study may have two treatment periods of 4 weeks each, with one washout week at the beginning and one in the middle. For a comparable parallel study, each subject will be in the trial for 5 weeks (one wash-out week plus four treatment weeks). The crossover study will clearly necessitate more subject visits, invariably more than they would make in the

The Institute of Clinical Research

normal course of treatment. This increases the probability of subjects dropping out, or even not entering. The visit schedule is clearly more of a burden and such considerations must be discussed with the prospective Investigator when planning the design.

The choice of a comparator for a crossover study must be made carefully. For example, the side-effect profile is an important factor. A crossover comparison between drugs with such different side-effect profiles as a beta-blocker (bradycardia) and a calcium entry blocker (tachycardia) may cause a double-blind study to become unblinded, therefore leading to the potential for bias.

Careful consideration of such issues will ensure that the crossover design is used in an appropriate way. Statistical advice is of paramount importance at the design phase, and the final analysis must investigate the possibility that differences observed between treatments may be due to 'period effects' rather than to genuine treatment differences.

In the clinical trial situation, the use of the crossover design may mean that the number of subjects in the study will be smaller than in a parallel design. See Statistics in Clinical Research[7] for a discussion of the issues of statistical power. This reduction in subject numbers is useful in some of the less prevalent diseases, or where time to trial completion is important.

Alternative trial designs

Ethics are a prime consideration in the design of clinical trials. It is a basic principle that no subject should be harmed by receiving a drug that is known to be inferior. Hence it may be considered appropriate in some instances to review the incoming data to avoid prolonging a trial where efficacy has been established beyond doubt. Analyses carried out to assess between-treatment differences while a trial is ongoing are called *interim analyses*. Interim analyses may not be as extensive as the final analysis, and may be based solely on safety reports.

There are major statistical complications to be overcome if interim analyses with significance testing are required in a trial. The use of repeated significance tests increases the chance of detecting a treatment difference at the conventionally accepted level of 5%, and the possibility of reporting a false- positive error is increased. As a consequence, a significance level that is more stringent than $p<0.05$ must be chosen. This will influence the sample size in the study, and statistical input is vital in this context. Most importantly, interim analyses should always be planned from the outset, and stopping rules should be developed at that time. Interim analyses are discussed further by Pocock[16].

Sequential design

A type of trial design that uses repeated analyses is the sequential design. With this design groups of subjects are studied in parallel, with analyses carried

The Institute of Clinical Research

out repeatedly, for example, after receipt of each subject's data, until a clear difference is shown between the treatments. Alternatively, it may become clear that no difference will be revealed. The advantage of this design is that the total trial length may be reduced, as fewer subjects would be needed. This type of trial is useful for rare diseases, particularly where a rapid response to treatment is likely to be shown by each subject. Certain practical problems are posed when planning a sequential trial with analysis after each subject. A group sequential design, where analysis is carried out after treatment of blocks of subjects, may be easier to conduct, particularly in a multicenter trial. The analyses must be carried out at predetermined intervals usually based on patient numbers until a difference is shown between treatments or it becomes clear that there is no difference. This design is ethically sound as the number of patients is reduced and the length of time in a trial is reduced[16]. As discussed before there are, however, statistical complications with interim analyses and multiplicity. There is also the added practical complication of multiple database locks.

Factorial design
Sometimes in a trial a comparison of a number of treatments is required. To complete multiple comparisons would require complex multiple arm parallel group designs or could result in the possibility of having to conduct several separate studies to evaluate each treatment. The factorial design allows evaluation of several treatments within the same trial by using various combinations of the treatments.

In a balanced 2 x 2 design of 12 patients, for example 6 receive intervention A, 6 are randomised to receive no intervention A. Correspondingly, 6 receive intervention B, or 6 do not receive intervention B.

Overall:
3 receive no intervention
3 receive intervention A only
3 receive intervention B only
3 receive A + B simultaneously

A greater number receives each treatment i.e. (50%) receive each treatment.

What are the advantages of a factorial design? A comparison of multiple treatments in a single study instead of separate studies is an advantage and fewer subjects are required than in multiple arm parallel trials. Factorial designs can study whether combinations of treatments are effective, it can identify the best dose of two treatments used together and can also evaluate interaction effects

For example, in order to find the best combination of treatments of A B C or placebo in an oncology trial, there are eight possible combinations:

A+B+C	A alone
A+B	B alone
A+C	C alone
B+C	neither A, B or C

Within-patient design

The crossover design is a type of within-patient comparison: a further design of this type is the within-patient comparison in which treatments are compared in the same subjects at the same time. This type of design will eliminate much of the variability, such as that due to timing of treatment, but its use is limited to treatments that may be administered to different parts of the anatomy independently. An example would be topical treatment of psoriasis in circumstances where there is no systemic absorption of the active compound.

A further variation on this type of design is the matched pair design where pairs of subjects are treated with the alternative treatments. The pairs will be matched for the age, sex and those prognostic factors appropriate to the indication[19].

Chapter Eight - Duration of dosing and clinical methods

Dosing

The factors that will determine the most appropriate duration of dosing and frequency of dosing are the pharmacokinetics and mode of action of the drug and the natural history of the disease being treated. However, beyond these clinical and scientific considerations there are many practical issues.

Particularly in early Phase II, available toxicology data may support only a limited duration of dosing. A drug development programme will include substantial chronic animal toxicology studies often running in parallel with the clinical phases, and results from these studies may extend the permissible duration of dosing as they become available. ICH M3 guideline[20] outlines the principles for the development of non-clinical strategies on the timing of toxicity studies in relation to the conduct of clinical trials. Consultation with the regulatory department will ensure that a study plan is within the regulations for clinical trials in the candidate countries. Some countries require a shorter period of animal dosing to support human dosing than others, and trials may be completed sooner by conducting them there, but the ethical requirement for adequate safety data must always be paramount.

Before designing a study of any length it is essential to ensure that sufficient supplies of the drug will be available. Any alteration of the dosing period may have far-reaching consequences; for example, an increase of the study period from 2 to 4 weeks doubles the amount of drug required. Consultation with the clinical trial supplies department is essential to ensure that the trial can be supported. This is particularly important in Phase II, at a time when the drug is not yet being manufactured in large quantities. Another issue concerning clinical trial supplies is the expiry date/retest date. At very early stages of development, the stability data for the test drug may provide only a short shelf-life and subjects may require new supplies. The visit schedule might have to accommodate visits for further supply, and the packaging should be planned to be synchronous with the supplies. This is a particular problem for trials with long treatment periods.

Methods of clinical measurement

The assessment method must be standardised so that the results from all subjects may be pooled and therefore the trial design will specify which method will be used and at what time intervals throughout the study. It may appear obvious to state that the measurement method chosen must be relevant, but in ensuring relevance, some factors listed below should be considered.

The method chosen must have been validated as being accurate and reproducible in the given situation. For a quantitative measurement such as blood pressure, the use of standardised calibrated equipment, e.g. the sphygmomanometer, is clearly most appropriate. For an assessment of a more subjective parameter, e.g. depression, there may be many rating scales available, or there may be proposals to use a new scale. In such a situation it is advisable to use a scale for which there is documented information about its specificity and reproducibility to provide an assessment of the depression. Without appropriate assurance of the validity of a new scale in the same population, it could be unwise to use any novel instrument to support claims of efficacy for a new treatment. It is advisable to use or develop new scales in parallel with established ones.

Assessment methods used for typical practice may not be appropriate for repeated use in clinical trials. This type of situation sometimes leads to the development of scales specifically for use in trials. For example, in the assessment of depression, standard rating scales such as the Hamilton Rating Scale for Depression were felt to lack sensitivity in consistently detecting differences between drugs. A new scale was therefore developed and validated for this purpose[22].

Having confirmed that the method is suitable for assessment of the given parameter, the practical feasibility of the measurement method must be addressed. The time required to carry out the measurement should be determined because outpatient visits may be brief. Frequent, repeated inpatient measurements may be very timeconsuming; for example, studies of analgesic efficacy following administration of a single dose will require the time of a devoted observer, or a subject in the immediate postoperative period may have difficulty responding. The statistical implications of such repeated measures such as this should also be considered[16].

The timing and circumstances of the assessment should be standardised when considering the design of a trial. Even the result of an apparently objective and quantitative measurement such as blood pressure will be influenced by circumstance unless a standard procedure is specified. For example, the subject should have been sitting for 10 minutes before two blood pressure readings are taken, and the mean of the two readings is then used for analysis. This type of instruction will control many of the biases caused by local circumstances. Additionally, the time of day for the measurement may be standardised to avoid the introduction of additional variability due to diurnal variation. There is a further cause of bias that can be controlled, namely observer bias. In the case of blood pressure, this may be due to number preferences, or 'rounding' when reading the pressure. The use of a device such as a random zero sphygmomanometer is one way to avoid this pitfall. The device introduces a random baseline, which is subtracted from the numbers initially recorded to obtain the true blood pressure.

The choice of measurement method will affect other aspects of the trial design because of the statistical implications. The accuracy of the measurement, reflected by the variability about the mean (SD), will be needed for the calculation of the sample size. Additionally, the statistician will require information about what is considered to be a clinically relevant difference according to the key measurement method. The sample size chosen should be such that, given the variability, a clinically relevant difference will be detected.

Regulatory authorities such as the European Medicines Agency (EMEA), Food and Drug Administration (FDA) and the World Health Organization (WHO) and ICH have published guidelines on preferred and acceptable clinical measurement techniques in many areas of drug development. Further useful information can be derived from European Public Assessment Reports (EPARs) if there has been a recent approval of a similar drug. An EPAR reflects the scientific conclusion reached by the Committee for Proprietary Medicinal Products (CPMP) at the end of the centralised evaluation process and provides a summary of the grounds for the CPMP opinion in favour of granting a marketing authorisation for a specific medicinal product. It is made available by the EMEA for information after deletion of commercially confidential information. In the US there are two ways of getting input to ensure acceptable trial design. A similar report to the EPAR is available as a Summary Basis of Approval (SBA), which details the basis of approval for marketed products. In addition Special Protocol Assessments (SPAs) provide an expedited evaluation by FDA of certain manufacturing, toxicology and clinical trial protocols to assess whether they are adequate to meet scientific and regulatory requirements. SPAs provide valuable information for Sponsors, significantly reducing regulatory uncertainty.

Chapter Nine - Other trial designs

The considerations thus far have dealt with the RCT but there are other trial designs that need to be considered

Epidemiology study designs

Epidemiology is the study of health and disease in populations including aetiology, natural course and treatments.

Cohort studies

Cohort studies are widely used in epidemiological research to investigate the incidence of events or disease and their cause. A prospective cohort study begins with the selection of a group of individuals who do not have the disease or outcome of interest. The individuals are then observed over a period of time to determine what happens to the patient and who develops the disease or outcome of interest.

Cohort studies are used to give a better understanding of the course of a disease, particularly referral patterns, resource use and long term adverse effects. An example of a cohort study is the British Doctors Study[23] to look at the aetiology factors for lung cancer. This large study in approximately 34,500 patients established a strong association between smoking and lung cancer. The cohort has been followed up for 40 years by means of questionnaires. Approximately 10,000 died in the first 20 years and a further 10,000 died during the following 20 years. The death rate ratio of smokers to non-smokers in the second 20-year period was threefold at ages 45-64 and twofold at 65-84. The interpretation of cohort data is improved by having a carefully selected control group where subjects can be matched for possible confounding variables where eligibility criteria and outcomes can be standardised.

This observational design is, however, open to over-enthusiasm and is prone to selection bias and losses to follow up. They are less suitable for establishing effectiveness but will detect associations but not necessarily causality. They do, however, give insight for answering questions on prognosis which is a feature of outcomes research.

Case-control studies

Another design associated with epidemiology is the case-control study. This design uses retrospective comparisons about aetiology of disease. Patients who have a disease are compared to those that do not have the disease with the aim of defining the relative contribution of one or several factors to the frequency of the disease.

Case-control studies are a less expensive and often use a type of epidemiological study which can be carried out by small teams or individual

The Institute of Clinical Research

researchers in single facilities, in a way which more structured trials often cannot. They are also ideal for investigating rare events since you start with the cases already identified. The success of these studies relies on rigorous case selection and well-matched controls.

They have pointed the way to a number of important discoveries and advances linking lung cancer, for example, with smoking history and asbestos exposure. Their very success has led some to place excessive faith in them to the point where their credibility has been significantly undermined. There have been links between vitamins and cancer; MMR and autism; antibiotics and asthma; cannabis and psychosis. All these have been identified through small-scale case-control studies but fail to show any effect in large scale RCTs. This is largely the result of misconceptions regarding the nature of such studies.

Outcomes research

Colleagues in different, but related, specialist disciplines now frequently demand that extra measurements be added into a trial. Examples include quality of life (QoL) assessments and pharmacoeconomics. There are advantages in including extra measurements into a study, as this might reduce the number of subjects who need to be treated, but it is unwise to attempt to achieve too much with a single trial. Extra measurements are often timeconsuming, and the clinical setting of the original trial may not be appropriate for gathering this additional information.

Traditionally the focus of clinical research has been on the endpoints employed to define success or failure of a treatment or intervention. Now, outcomes of a new drug or intervention, is considered more broadly looking at changes in patient quality of life but also on the health service in terms of numbers of inpatient days in hospital.

Outcomes research looks not only at the efficacy of a treatment or intervention i.e. does a treatment work in ideal conditions, but also looks at effectiveness, i.e. does it work in normal practice?

Quality of life (QoL)

In response to the increasing demands of governmental health care policies worldwide, the pharmaceutical industry is investigating the impact of new treatments on aspects other than disease severity. The assessment of QoL is becoming common and may be used to identify benefits of one treatment over another when their effect on the disease is equal. These studies measure the physical, emotional and social aspects of an illness and its treatment. A treatment that improves clinical status but reduces QoL may not be a positive outcome, but a treatment that has little effect on illness severity but improved QoL may be useful to patients. An example of this may be the comparison of a beta-blocker and an angiotensin-converting enzyme (ACE) inhibitor in

The Institute of Clinical Research

the treatment of high blood pressure. The two do not differ to any clinically significant extent in terms of lowering blood pressure, but subjects receiving th ACE inhibitor feel better. QoL assessment scales have been developed to assess what 'feeling better' means, in an attempt to quantify apparently subjective endpoints. In some cases the scale may identify which drug displays the most acceptable adverse effect profile.

As with all measurement methods, the scale chosen must be appropriate for the situation; it should be meaningful for the disease being studied, and should be practical to administer in the given trial situation. There are a number of quality of life scales, some disease specific like EORTIC QOQ[24] for cancer and some generic like SF-36[25]. QoL scales can be added to pivotal studies, e.g. we may reduce the blood pressure, but do we reduce stroke or heart disease or does the patient experience adverse events? The benefit of treatment may be measured in QALYs (Quality Adjusted Life Years), which combines both quality and quantity of life.

Pharmacoeconomic studies

Pharmacoeconomics is a field that has grown in response to pricing policies of health care purchasers, usually governments. The cost of pharmaceuticals is an obvious target for price control, as the other elements of health care are not so clearly defined. Hence, the need to demonstrate the benefits achieved by a new treatment in relation to cost, as well as the savings made elsewhere in the health care process or in society at large. Pharmacoeconomic studies allow comparison of health resource implications as they do not focus just on the efficacy of a drug but also effects on the length of hospital stay, doctors' time, the use of hospital beds and on consequences for example avoidance of an event such as heart attack.

There are four main types of study:

Cost effectiveness, which examines the cost of treating a patient. If you compare two antibiotics the outcome can be measured in the same way (number of infections resolved by the antibiotics) and the costs expressed as cost per unit outcome i.e. cost per infection resolved.

Cost minimisation, is a form of cost-effectiveness analysis where benefits have been proven (assumed) to be equal. It measures cost alone so you choose the cheapest treatment. If you compare a branded drug versus a generic drug the decision is made on least cost, i.e. the generic drug.

Cost benefit, compares the costs of treatments with the effects measured in money. Allows comparison across all treatments because effects are measured in the same units and can tell us whether a treatment is worthwhile (i.e. whether benefit outweighs cost). The outcome is the saving made by comparing different treatments, i.e. cost consequence.

Cost utility, is a comparative analysis of alternative courses of action, it focuses particular attention on the quality of the health outcome. QALYs - unit of output that combines both quality and quantity of life (QoL). These studies measure the value in terms of value derived from the treatment by the patient comparing the cost per QALY of each treatment. This economic evaluation is useful when a health authority has to choose in which patient groups to spend scarce resources or money, e.g. hip replacement or heart transplant.

Increasingly companies and academia have to demonstrate economic evaluation of a treatment and more Phase III and IV studies include such assessments. Outcome research, which encompasses clinical, economic and social outcomes of treatment is becoming increasingly important with the possibility of a European body being set up to evaluate economic analysis alongside clinical trials.

Pharmacokinetic sampling/dose escalation/dose response

The single escalating dose study is commonly used in Phase I development. The starting dose in man is calculated based on 1% or 2% of the No Observable Adverse Effect Level (NOAEL) dose in animals. Vaidya suggest, using the following three different methods for evolving a starting dose in Phase I studies:

- 10-20% of the maximum tolerated dose in the most sensitive species of animal tested

- Examination of animal data to assess the dose which produces the pharmacodynamic action relevant for its proposed therapeutic role in man

- Scrutiny of the effective and safe does in man of closely related compounds.

Often 8-12 volunteers are used. 2-4 receive placebo and 6-8 receive the test drug. Screening is usually carried out within 2-4 weeks before drug administration. Meticulous screening is carried out to minimise risk and facilitate interpretation of results. The drug is then given and blood and urine samples are taken at various time points according to the kinetic properties predicted from preclinical work. The next group of volunteers should not receive the drug until the results of the previous group safety tests are known. The doses in each group may be increased by doubling doses used in the previous stage or by smaller or larger steps. The increments are stopped by the appearance of toxicity or attainment of the desired activity. The route of administration should be the intended market route (usually oral administration) which is safer cheaper and more convenient than injections. No route of administration that has not been previously tested in animals should be used.

Repeated administration

Only when single dose administration has been investigated, can multiple dose studies begin. In this type of study, drug or placebo is given repeatedly for one or more weeks but it is dependent on disease area. Antibiotics for example may be tested for a shorter period of 5-7 days whereas an anticonvulsant (which is likely to be used for several years) may be tested for 4 weeks or more in Phase I. The interval between doses is usually one half-life but it is desirable to aim at what can be easily accomplished once a day, twice a day, etc.

In designing Phase II and Phase III trials, the pharmacokinetics of the test treatment will be known. However, the early pharmacokinetic studies will have been conducted intensively in small numbers of subjects who are often healthy volunteers but sometimes patients. In parallel with broadening the target population for the safety and efficacy assessments, so that Phase III closely approximates to the target population, there has been a recent development in pharmacokinetics known as population pharmacokinetics.

The aim of population pharmacokinetics is to collect a small number of samples for drug concentration assay from a large number of subjects, in order to identify the extent of variability in the population. This may have implications, for example, in dosing. Basic demographic details of the subjects need to be recorded: age, weight, race and, depending on the type of drug, metabolic status. The samples, perhaps only two or three, would be collected at target times associated with one dose. The modelling of the pharmacokinetic parameters will take account of variability around the target times, but the accurate times in relation to a dose must be recorded.

The incorporation of such testing into a trial design should ensure that it does not interfere with the primary objective, which is probably an efficacy assessment. Additionally, it must be practically feasible. This type of sampling may be carried out in long-term studies, and if the subjects are outpatients, or the trial is carried out in a general practice setting, the availability of adequate time and facilities should be ensured.

Chapter Ten - Multicentre trials

Designing a multicentre trial

The need to increase the number of subjects who have received a new treatment prior to marketing approval, combined with the need to study these increased numbers in a limited time, means that many trials, in particular in Phase III, will be carried out at more than one centre. Such trials are called multicentre trials. The aim of this chapter so far has been to discuss ways of avoiding or controlling bias in the results of a trial by carefully choosing the elements in its design. The introduction of more than one investigational site multiplies the ways in which bias can be introduced. Some of the elements discussed above will be readdressed here to highlight points that will require additional consideration when several people are involved, not only at the investigational site but also in the Sponsor organisation.

Multicentre trials may be carried out in one country only, or in more than one. The multinational, multicentre trial has been chosen for this discussion.

Choice of comparator

In cases where an active comparator is necessary for the study, it must be one that is registered in all the target countries, both for the indication required and at the same dosage. This is not always the case. Advice from regulatory experts will be necessary to investigate ways of overcoming any restrictions that a lack of standardisation may impose. Packaging and formulation may also need to be reviewed carefully to ensure that the study will comply with regulations in all countries. Differences in clinical practice are more difficult to tackle than these regulatory issues. For example, the standard treatment in one country may not be considered efficacious or safe in another, and is therefore disqualified from use as a standard comparator.

The placebo-controlled trial

There will undoubtedly be as many different views about the suitability of a placebo-controlled trial as there are centres in the study. Therefore, the ethical issues must be clearly addressed in the earliest stages of study preparation.

Patient population

Differences in clinical practice may emerge when discussing the population of study participants. There may be differing opinions as to what defines a particular disease, and also what severity of disease demands which type of treatment. Clarity in defining the study population is most important. This may require prolonged discussion in order to identify sufficient numbers of subjects according to a common definition.

The Institute of Clinical Research

Concurrent diseases and concomitant medication

While concurrent diseases may be easy to control by excluding certain subjects, the use of concomitant medication is difficult to standardise. Different formulations and different dosage regimens will be used, and often entirely different treatments. To address this issue, it must be clear what influence any concomitant medication will have on the primary objective of the study. In certain situations it may be impossible to change a hospital protocol that is well established and used by all staff members. A most valuable way to resolve clinical differences is to arrange a meeting of the Investigators to discuss ways to compromise, where necessary.

Clinical measurement

The use of clinical measurement methods must be standardised at all centres. An example will serve to illustrate how detailed the instructions must be. While a tape measure may be used to record the circumference of a swollen ankle, each individual may take the measurement at a slightly different place. Therefore, the distance from the tibial tubercle to the measurement point, and the position of the subject, should be specified. To avoid diurnal variation, the time of day of measurement should be stipulated. To control for environmental factors, the weather, or the fact that the subject was driven to the clinic rather than driving him/herself, the uninjured ankle is also measured, and the difference between the two is used in the analysis. This may seem a long 'protocol' for something relatively simple, but it is necessary to achieve standardisation. For subjective assessment methods there are even more sources of potential inconsistency. The way that a question is asked will influence the answer, even within one culture. When this is extended to a multinational study, many problems arise. This is also related to language. The example of a four-point verbal rating scale of 'none', 'mild', 'moderate' and 'severe' may produce a different distribution of results across Europe. Rating scales may be validated in the language for which they were developed, but for use in another language they must first be translated, and then validated again, because the subtleties of the assessment may be lost in a different language or culture.

Chapter Eleven - Evidence-based medicine (EBM)

No monograph on the design of clinical trials is complete without consideration of evidence-based medicine. The Centre for Evidence Based Medicine (CEBM) states 'evidence based medicine is the integration of best research evidence with clinical expertise and patient values'[27].

Best research evidence means clinically relevant research, often from the basic sciences of medicine, but especially from patient centred clinical research into the accuracy and precision of diagnostic tests (including the clinical examination), the power of prognostic markers, and the efficacy and safety of therapeutic, rehabilitative, and preventive regimens. New evidence from clinical research both invalidates previously accepted diagnostic tests and treatments and replaces them with new ones that are more powerful, more accurate, more efficacious, and safer.

Clinical expertise means the ability to use clinical skills and past experience to rapidly identify each patient's unique health state and diagnosis, their individual risks and benefits of potential interventions, and their personal values and expectations.

Patient values are the unique preferences, concerns and expectations each patient brings to a clinical encounter and which must be integrated into clinical decisions if they are to serve the patient.

When these three elements are integrated, clinicians and patients form a diagnostic and therapeutic alliance, which optimises clinical outcomes and quality of life.

The next step would be to determine the best study design needed to answer the clinical question.

There are four categories of EBM questions:

- **Therapy:** solves questions about which treatment to administer, and what might be the outcome of different treatment options. For most therapy questions one may want to look for the best evidence namely a randomised controlled study, and if the study is double blind it is more robust. Example: find the evidence for the use of anticoagulants in patients with atrial fibrillation.

- **Diagnosis:** solves questions about the degree to which a test is reliable and clinically useful, to decide whether the patient would benefit from it. Most articles compare the results of a certain diagnostic test with that of a standard test regarded as being a 'gold standard'. Example: search for the best diagnostic test for Alzheimer's disease.

- **Aetiology:** solves problems about the relationship between a disease and a possible cause. Example: find out if a diet rich in saturated fats increases the risk of heart disease, and if so by how much.

- **Prognosis:** answers questions about a patient's future health, life span and quality of life in the event one chooses a particular treatment option. Example: find how the quality of life would change for a patient who undergoes surgery for prostate cancer.

Certain study designs are superior to others when answering particular questions. RCTs are considered the best for addressing questions about therapy, whereas other study designs are appropriate for addressing other types of questions e.g. aetiology questions may be addressed by case-control and cohort studies. Other aspects relevant to study design include placebo comparison group and follow-up.

- Randomized controlled trial - answers therapy, prevention questions

- Cohort study - answers prognosis, aetiology, prevention questions

- Case control study - answers prognosis, aetiology, prevention questions.

- Case series and case reports - answers prognosis, aetiology, prevention questions.

The strength of a study depends on its design.

A hierarchy of evidence exists with decreasing strength as follows:

- Systematic review and meta-analysis

- Randomised controlled trials with definitive results

- Randomised controlled trials with non-definitive results

- Cohort studies

- Case-control studies

- Cross-sectional surveys

- Case reports.

The emergence of new types of evidence being generated can create changes in the way patients are treated. Clinicians who keep up to date with these advances in knowledge practice better medicine. Unfortunately, given the extremely rapid growth of randomised trials and other rigorous clinical investigations, the issue is no longer how little of medical practice has a firm basis in such evidence, the issue today is how much of what is firmly based is actually applied in patient care.

The clinical literature is now so big that general physicians who want to keep abreast of the journals relevant to their practices have to examine 19 articles a day, 365 days a year[28].

One of the fundamental skills required for practising EBM is asking well-thought out clinical questions. To benefit patients and clinicians, such questions need to be both directly relevant to patients' problems and phrased in ways that direct a search to relevant and precise answers. In practice, well-thought out clinical questions usually contain four elements: patient, intervention, comparison of intervention and outcomes (PICO, Table 3)[29].

	1 Patient or Problem	2 Intervention (a cause, prognostic factor, treatment etc)	3 Comparison Intervention (if necessary)	4 Outcomes
Tips for Building	Starting with your patient, ask 'How would I describe a group of patients similar to mine?' Balance precision with brevity.	Ask "Which main intervention am I considering?" Be specific.	Ask "What is the main alternative to compare with the intervention?" Again, be specific.	Ask "What can I accomplish?" or "What could this exposure really affect?" Again, be specific.
Example	'In patients with heart failure from dilated cardiomyopathy, who are in sinus rhythm	"... would adding anticoagulation with warfarin to standard failure therapy ..."	"... when compared with standard therapy alone ..."	"... lead to lower mortality or morbidity from thromboembolism. Is this enough to be worth the increased risk of bleeding?"

Once a question is formulated using the PICO structure, the question being asked points to the type of research that would provide the best answer. Critical appraisal is the process of deciding whether a piece of research can help in answering a clinical question. There are three questions to ask about any kind of research:

- Is it valid?
- Is it important?
- Is it applicable to the patient?

Clearly, different kinds of research are different in terms of methodological validity, how they present their results and how they translate to an individual patient. There are a number of tools available to help researchers appraise the information in literature, e.g. CAT[29].

In selecting treatments for patients, until recently it was considered sufficient to understand the pathophysiological process in a disorder and to prescribe drugs or other treatments that had been shown to interrupt or modify this process.

For example, the observation that patients with ventricular ectopic beats following myocardial infarction were seen to be at high risk of sudden death. However, subsequent randomised controlled trials examined hard clinical outcomes, not physiological processes, and showed that several of these drugs increase, rather than decrease, the risk of death in such patients, and their routine use is now strongly discouraged.

In order for EBM to arrive at the most appropriate conclusion about a therapy, all available evidence must be reviewed. The most important evidence is derived from RCT and therefore it is imperative that such studies are designed to meet the appropriate standards.

The
Institute
of
Clinical
Research

Chapter Twelve - Reporting and publishing data

Clinical trials are one of the most important sources of scientific evidence on the safety and effectiveness of health interventions. Access to information about ongoing, completed and published clinical trials is essential for appropriate decision-making.

Any clinical trial that is conducted for an MAA will be written up in the form of a clinical trial report. The format and content of the report is described in the guideline ICH E3[30]. The guideline outlines the compilation of a single core clinical study report acceptable to all regulatory authorities of the ICH regions. The regulatory authority specific additions will consist of modules to be considered as appendices, available upon request according to regional regulatory requirements.

The guideline is intended to assist Sponsors in the development of a report that is complete, free from ambiguity, well organised and easy to review. The report should provide a clear explanation of how the critical design features of the study were chosen and enough information on the plan, methods and conduct of the study so that there is no ambiguity in how the study was carried out. The report with its appendices should also provide enough individual patient data, including the demographic and baseline data, and details of analytical methods, to allow replication of the critical analyses when authorities wish to do so.

Although clinical reports are written the results are not always published.

It is apparent that published clinical trial data do not always represent the true extent of research being undertaken. People involved in research including Investigators, Sponsors and editors typically prefer positive trial outcomes. Trials generating negative or unequivocal results are less likely to be published in peer review journals and this can undermine the integrity of clinical research data. The lack of interest in publishing non-positive results might at least be partly due to underpowered studies. In such trials results become indeterminate which makes them of no interest to journal editors.

The publicity associated with Glaxo SmithKline's antidepressant Paxil/Seroxat increased concerns about marketing practices and the conduct of clinical trials and disclosure of results[31]. One way of preventing such publication bias is by introducing compulsory registration of trials at initiation and ensuring that all results of all trials are published.

In its effort to develop worldwide standards of trial registration, the World Health Organization (WHO) launched its International Clinical Trials Registry Platform (ICTRP)[32] project. The project is 'taking the lead in setting international norms and standards for trial registration and reporting.'

The Institute of Clinical Research

Transparency in research and knowledge sharing are now widely seen as a precondition for the success of health research. Trial registries are an important tool to help achieve this transparency. The Internet has made electronic registries entirely feasible. The vision of freely accessible electronic depositories of protocol information of ongoing trials and their results, with each trial assigned a unique number so that it can be tracked, is now achievable. In the EU such data although not freely available, is possible by means of the EudraCT database[33]. A register of completed and mostly published trials has been compiled by the Cochrane Collaboration and is regularly updated, but it is not as complete as it could be[34].

Many registries have been developed to meet various specific needs. One of these registries is the International Standard Randomized Controlled Trial Number (ISRCTN) register, run by the National Library of Medicine (NLM)[35]. The WHO, the Ottawa Group, and the International Committee of Medical Journal Editors (ICMJE) although starting from different points, and having some different specific goals, overlap on the important registration premise to provide free electronic access (open access) to deposited, essential information of ongoing trials. It is important that standards for universal trial registration be defined and applied globally.

There is clearly a need for change leading to research based on transparency, full disclosure, and collaboration and although protection of commercial interests is important, publishers, clinicians and patients alike need to check whether they are getting the full picture when they are provided with 'evidence' for new treatments.

Chapter Thirteen - Summary

The importance of appropriate clinical trial design cannot be overestimated because every element in a clinical trial is influenced by its design. Every study team member should have a role in design development. Poor planning at the design stage can result in costly R&D losses, in terms both of budget and resource. Marketing pressures should not be allowed to compromise careful and timely consideration of trial design.

Every effort must be made to ensure that the clinical trial is consistent with its scientific objective and is not open to criticism because of poor design.

Clinical trials are one of the most important sources of scientific evidence on the safety and effectiveness of health interventions. Poorly designed and conducted trials can lead to misleading information on clinical outcomes and the quality of life of patients.

At the time of writing, the impact of genetic research on clinical research, and therefore on clinical trial design, is unclear but inevitable. Knowledge acquired through genomics may enable us to predict more clearly which subjects are likely to benefit from certain classes of drug, and which subjects are likely to experience side effects. The implication may be that subjects selected to participate in clinical trials will display less variability, while this may lead to a reduction in subject numbers required, it may also have an impact on the generality of the data obtained. However, genetic material is being collected for future research, but genomics is still in its infancy and has to clear a number of hurdles (e.g. ethics) before any radical changes can take place.

References

1   ICH Secretariat Topic E6 Good Clinical Practice, Step 5: Consolidated Guideline 1 May 1996, CPMP/ICH/135/95

2   ICH Secretariat Topic E8 General Considerations for Clinical Trials, Step 5, September 97, issued as CPMP/ICH/291/95

3   The European Parliament and Council, Directive 2001/20/EC on the approximation of the laws, regulations and administration provisions of the Member States relating to the implementation of good clinical practice in the conduct of clinical trials on medicinal products for human use, 4 April 2001

4   The European Parliament and Council, Directive 2005/28/EC laying down principles and detailed guidelines for good clinical practice as regards investigational medicinal products for human use, as well as the requirements for authorisation of the manufacturing or importation of such products, 8 April 2005

5   ICH Secretariat Topic E4 Dose-Response Information to Support Drug Registration, Step 5, May 94, issued as CPMP/ICH/378/95

6   ICH Secretariat Topic E10 Choice of Control Group in Clinical Trials, Step 5, 20 July 2000, CPMP/ICH/364/96

7   Parry T, Parrott A (ed) (2004). Statistics in Clinical Research, The Institute of Clinical Research

8   FDA, 21 CFR part 314, Applications for FDA approval to market a new drug, 1 April 2003

9   Hrobjartsson A, Gotzsche P (2001). Is the placebo powerless? An analysis of clinical trials comparing placebo with no treatment. *N Engl J Med* 344: 1594–1602

10 WMA, Ethical Principles for Medical Research Involving Human Subjects (Declaration of Helsinki) Tokyo 2004, other versions 2002, 2000, 1996, 1989

11 Weihrauch, TR and Gauler, TC (1999). Placebo-efficacy and adverse effects in controlled clinical trials. *Arzneimittelforschung* 49, 385-393

12 McQuay HJ, Bullingham RES, Moore RA, Evans PJD, Lloyd JW (1982). Some patients don't need analgesics after surgery. J *Roy Soc Med* 75,705-708

13 Dumville JC, Hahn S, Miles JNV and Torgerson DJ (2006). The use of unequal randomisation ratios in clinical trials: a review. *Contemporary Clinical Trials* 27 (2006) 1–12

14 Fitzpatrick S, Downes N (ed) (2005). The Clinical Trial Protocol, The Institute of Clinical Research

15 Kernan WN, Viscoli CM, Makuch RW, Brass LM, Horwitz RI (1999). Stratified randomization for clinical trials. J *Clin Epidemiol* 52, 19-26

16 Pocock SJ (1983). *Clinical Trials: A Practical Approach.* John Wiley, Chichester

17 Nguyen M, Kabir M and Ravaud P (2004). Short-term efficacy and safety of Leflunomide in the treatment of active rheumatoid arthritis in everyday clinical use. Clin Drug Invest 24(2):103-112

18 Palmer CR and Rosenberger WF (1999). Ethics and practice: alternative designs for Phase III randomized clinical trials. *Controlled Clinical Trials* 20, 172-186

19 Altman DO (1991). *Practical Statistics for Medical Research.* Chapman & Hall, London

20 ICH Secretariat Topic M3(R1):Maintenance of the ICH Guideline on Non-Clinical Safety Studies for the Conduct of Human Clinical Trials for Pharmaceuticals Step 5 in November 2000, CPMP/ICH286/95 modification

21 Hamilton M (1967). Development of a rating scale for primary depressive illness. *Br J Soc Clin Psychol* 6, 278-296

22 Montgomery SA, Asberg M (1979). A new depression scale designed to be sensitive to change. *Br J Psychiatry* 134, 382-38

23 Doll R, Peto R, Boreham J, Sutherland I, (2004). Mortality in relation to smoking: 50 years' observations on male British doctors *BMJ, doi:10.1136/ bmj.38142.554479.AE*

24 Blazeby J, Cull A, Groenvold M, Bottomley A. (2001). Guidelines for developing Quality of Life Questionnaires (Second Edition). *EORTC Quality of Life Group, Brussels*

25 Ware JE, Sherbourne CD (1992). The MOS 36-item Short-Form Health Survey (SF-36): I.Conceptual framework and item selection. *Medical Care:* 30: 473-83.SF36

26 Vaidya AB, Vaidya RA (1981). Initial human trials with an investigational new drug: planning and management J Post Grad Med 27. 197-213

27   http://www.cebm.net/ [accessed 5 July 2006]

28 Davidoff F, Haynes B, Sackett D, Smith R (1995). Evidence based medicine: a new journal to help doctors identify the information they need. *BMJ*;310: 1085-6.

29 Centre for Evidence-Based Medicine, http://www.cebm.net/focus_quest.asp [accessed 5 July 2006]

30 ICH Secretariat Topic E3 Structure and Content of Clinical Study Reports, Step 4, 30 November 1995, CPMP/ICH/137/95

31 Dyer O (2004). GlaxoSmithKline to set up comprehensive online clinical trials register. *BMJ* 329: 590-1

32 World Health Organization (2005). World Health Organization international clinical trials registry platform: Unique ID assignment. Geneva: World Health Organization. Available: http://www.who.int/ictrp/comments2/en/index.html. Accessed 20 September 2005

33 http://eudract.emea.eu.int/ [accessed 25 July 2006]

34 The Cochrane Collaboration http://www.cochrane.org/ [accessed 5 July 2006]

35 National Library of Medicine (NLM) http://www.nlm.nih.gov/ [accessed 5 July 2006]